The Great Smoothie Rush

Go Green and Lose Weight with these
Smoothies Recipes

By

Heston Brown

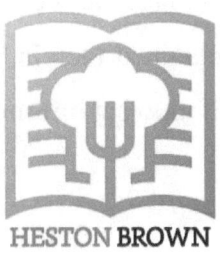

HESTON **BROWN**

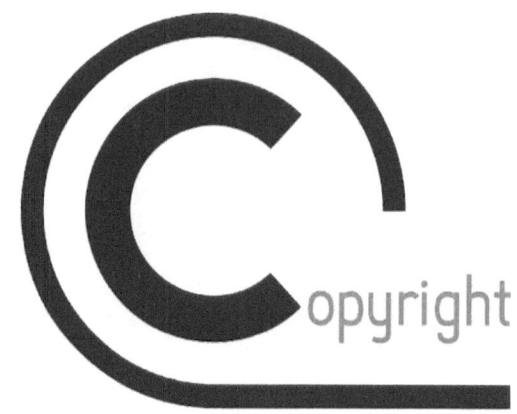

Copyright 2019 Heston Brown

Thank you so much for buying my book! I want to give you a special gift!

Receive a special gift as a thank you for buying my book. Now you will be able to benefit from free and discounted book offers that are sent directly to your inbox every week.

To subscribe simply fill in the box below with your details and start reaping the rewards! A new deal will arrive every day and reminders will be sent so you never miss out. Fill in the box below to subscribe and get started!

https://heston-brown.getresponsepages.com

Subscribe
to our
newsletter

Your Email

Table of Contents

Chapter I – Fat Burning Smoothies

xxxxxxxxxxxxxxxxxxxxxxxxxxxxxxxxxx

Natural fruits and vegetables have the ability to quickly burn your body fat. If you want to reduce weight, there are a few smoothies that are really delicious for everyone:

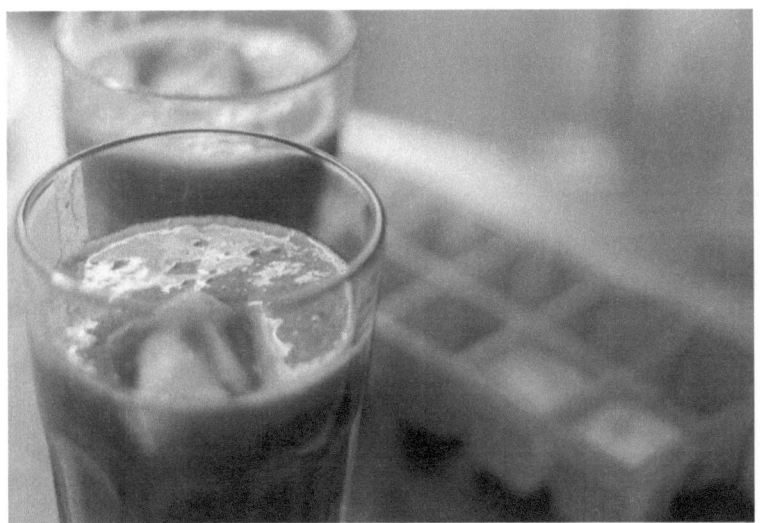

Recipe 1: Coconut and Raspberry Smoothie

Nutritional Importance: This smoothie is loaded with quercetin, gallic acid, vitamin C and other antioxidants. It is good to fight with obesity, cancer, heart diseases and age-related problems.

Preparation Time: 5 Minutes

Yield: 1 to 2 smoothies

List of Ingredients:

- Coconut milk: 1 cup
- Banana (remove peels and cut into slices): 1 medium
- Coconut extract: 2 tsp.
- Frozen raspberries: 1 cup
- Coconut flakes (shredded): As per taste

XXXXXXXXXXXXXXXXXXXXXXXXXXXXXXXXX

Methods:

Add milk, coconut extracts and banana slices to a blender. Pulse these ingredients for 1 to 2 minutes to make them smooth. Now, add raspberries in this blend and pulse them again to make them smooth. Pour into serving glasses and top with shredded coconut and raspberries. Enjoy!

Recipe 2: Chocolate and Cashew Butter

Nutritional Importance: This delicious smoothie is loaded with healthy fats, amino acids and dietary minerals. Make sure to carefully add cashew butter because extra use of this butter can increase its calorie count.

Preparation Time: 5 Minutes

Yield: 2 smoothies

List of Ingredients:

- Banana: 1
- Almond milk (unsweetened): 1 cup
- Cashew butter: 1 Tbsp.
- Dark chocolate (unsweetened): 1 packet or cocoa powder (2 Tbsp.)
- Vanilla extract: ½ tsp.
- Protein powder: 1 Tbsp. (optional)
- Ice: handful

XXXXXXXXXXXXXXXXXXXXXXXXXXXXXXXXXXX

Methods:

Combine all of these ingredients in a blender and blend them to make a smooth paste. Serve cold.

Recipe 3: Avocado and Spinach Smoothie

Nutritional Importance: This smoothie is loaded with monounsaturated fatty acids, fiber, potassium and other essential nutrients. It is good to reduce weight and cholesterol level in your body.

Preparation Time: 5 Minutes

Yield: 2 smoothies

List of Ingredients:

- Avocado (pitted and chopped): 1
- Fresh spinach: 1 cup
- Banana (ripe): 1
- Peanut butter: 1 Tbsp.
- Coconut milk: 1 cup
- Ice cubes: handful

xxxxxxxxxxxxxxxxxxxxxxxxxxxxxxxxxx

Methods:

Initially, blend avocado and spinach to make a smooth paste. Now, add rest of the ingredients and blend them again. Make sure to avoid any artificial sweetener and sugar.

Recipe 4: Pumpkin Smoothie with Chai Tea

Nutritional Importance: To detoxify your body, you can enjoy this smoothie in breakfast and even in the evening. This smoothie is loaded with calcium, copper, phosphorus, fiber, mono-unsaturated fatty acids, protein, vitamins and minerals.

Preparation Time: 5 Minutes

Yield: 2 smoothies

List of Ingredients:

- Almond milk (without sugar): 2/3 cup
- Vanilla: 1 tsp.
- Pumpkin pie (spice): ½ tsp.
- Chai tea (teabag): 1 tsp.
- Bananas: 2 frozen
- Pumpkin puree: 3 Tbsp.

xxxxxxxxxxxxxxxxxxxxxxxxxxxxxxxxxxx

Methods:

You have to combine all these ingredients (except banana) into one blender and blend them well to break down tea and other ingredients. If you are using loose leaves of tea, there is no problem because it can be easily broken down. If you are using a teabag, you can simply open the teabag and pour tea into a blender.

Once the mixture is blended, you have to add bananas and blend them for a few minutes. The Delicious smoothie is ready, but if you find it too thick, you can add extra milk and blend for one minute. Serve cold.

Recipe 5: Breakfast Smoothie with Berries and Oats

Nutritional Importance: Antioxidants in this smoothie will help your body to fight with oxidative stress often caused by free radicals and lead you to illness.

Preparation Time: 5 Minutes

Yield: 2 smoothies

List of Ingredients:

- Rolled oats: ½ cup
- Almond milk: 1 cup
- Frozen berries (or fresh): ½ cup
- Honey: 3 Tbsp.
- Greek yogurt: 1/3 cup
- Ice: ¼ cup

xxxxxxxxxxxxxxxxxxxxxxxxxxxxxxxxx

Methods:

Take a blender and one by one add all ingredients in this blender and blend them. Make sure to avoid any artificial sweetener and sugar. You can add extra milk to decrease its thickness. Serve immediately. You can use a combination of blackberries, strawberries, and raspberries.

Chapter II – Delicious Green Smoothies

xxxxxxxxxxxxxxxxxxxxxxxxxxxxxxxx

Green smoothies are rich in fiber, vitamin, iron and various other essential nutrients. There are recipes and health benefits of a few green smoothies:

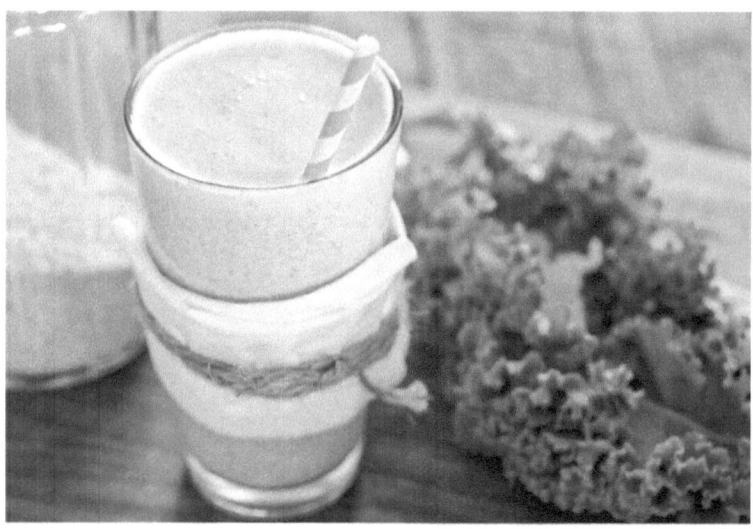

Recipe 1: Green Skin Cleanser

Nutritional Importance: Antioxidants in this smoothie can repair your damaged body tissues and skin cells. One glass of green smoothie is loaded with zinc, vitamins E and A. You can use it as a tonic to enhance your beauty.

Preparation Time: 5 Minutes

Yield: 2 smoothies

List of Ingredients:

- Fresh Spinach: 1 ½ cups
- Coconut water (without sweetness): 1 cup
- Pineapple (frozen): 1 cup
- Avocado (corded and chopped): ¼
- Ice cubes: 3 to 4

xxxxxxxxxxxxxxxxxxxxxxxxxxxxxxxxxx

Methods:

Initially, blend coconut milk and spinach to make a smooth paste. Now, add leftover ingredients and blend them once again to make a smooth blend. Enjoy cold.

Recipe 2: Vegetable Cocktail

Nutritional Importance: This cocktail can be an excellent replacement of one meal because fiber and many nutrients in this cocktail will keep you full for a longer period of time. It is good to cleanse your body.

Preparation Time: 5 Minutes

Yield: 2 smoothies

List of Ingredients:

- Kale (remove stems): 2 cups
- Tomatoes (chopped): 3 cups
- Celery rib: 1
- Sliced scallions: 2
- Minced garlic: ¼ tsp.
- Lime juice: 1 lime
- Red pepper (ground): 1/8 tsp.
- Salt: 1 pinch

xxxxxxxxxxxxxxxxxxxxxxxxxxxxxxxxxx

Methods:

Initially, blend tomatoes and kale to make a smooth paste. Now, add lime juice, celery, garlic, red pepper, salt and scallions to blend them again. Pour smoothie into your glasses, garnish glasses with a lemon slice and Enjoy cold.

Recipe 3: Coconut Green Smoothie

Nutritional Importance: This smoothie is a unique combination of essential fatty acids and has lots of positive effects on your health. This will help you to reduce fat, improve brain function and heart health.

Preparation Time: 5 Minutes

Yield: 2 smoothies

List of Ingredients:

- Clementine (remove peels and strings): 4 to 5
- Banana (sliced): 1 ripe
- Coconut milk: ½ cup
- Greens: 1 big handful
- Ice cubes: 3 to 4
- Mint leaves

xxxxxxxxxxxxxxxxxxxxxxxxxxxxxxxxxxx

Methods:

Take a blender and add every ingredient in this blender. Blend these ingredients to get a smooth and creamy blend. You can adjust flavors as per your needs, such as banana or a few mango slices for sweetness, herbs for earthiness and ice to make your smoothie thick.

Recipe 4: Tropical Green Blend with Mango

Nutritional Importance: This smoothie is packed with vitamins C, iron, magnesium, folate, magnesium and various other nutrients. This smoothie can keep you hydrated for a whole day.

Preparation Time: 5 Minutes

Yield: 2 smoothies

List of Ingredients:

- Fresh Spinach: 2 cups
- Orange (peeled): 1
- Coconut water (unsweetened): 1 cup
- Pineapple (frozen): 1 cup
- Frozen mango: 2 cups
- Lime juice: ½ lime
- A few slices of lemon to garnish

xxxxxxxxxxxxxxxxxxxxxxxxxxxxxxxxxxxx

Methods:

Initially, blend coconut milk and spinach to make a smooth paste. Now, add lime juice, pineapple and mango to blend them again. Pour smoothie in your glasses, garnish glasses with lemon slice and Enjoy cold.

Recipe 5: Tropical Green Smoothie

Health Benefits: Green smoothie is high in fiber, low in calories and zero in fats. It is filled with folate, vitamins, nutrients, iron and magnesium.

Preparation Time: 5 Minutes

Yield: 2 smoothies

List of Ingredients:

- Almond Milk: ¾ cups
- Bananas (remove peels and cut into slices): 2
- Pineapple chunks (fresh): 2 cups
- Kale: 2 cups

XXXXXXXXXXXXXXXXXXXXXXXXXXXXXXXXX

Methods:

Take a powerful blender and add all ingredients in this blender. Blend these ingredients for a few minutes at high speed to get a smooth and creamy blend. Use a scraper to scrape down all sides of blender as per your needs. If the smoothie is too thick, you can add extra milk. You can store leftover smoothie in the refrigerator for almost 8 to 10 hours.

Chapter III – Smoothies to Nourish Your Brain

xxxxxxxxxxxxxxxxxxxxxxxxxxxxxxxxxx

If you want to get extra energy and improve the overall health of your brain, you can get the advantage of these smoothies:

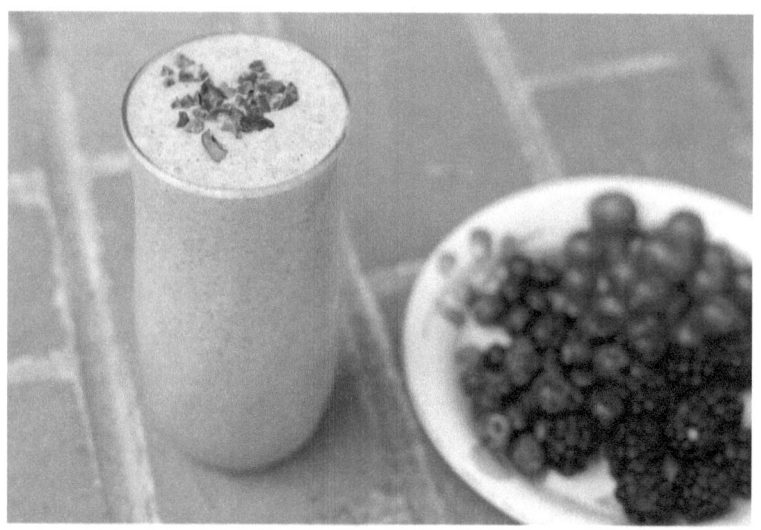

Recipe 1: Almond and Banana Smoothie

Nutritional Importance: Combination of banana and almond will be great to improve the overall health of your brain. Almonds are loaded with protein and dopamine. If you want to increase energy, you can get the advantage of this smoothie:

Preparation Time: 5 Minutes

Yield: 1 Smoothie

List of Ingredients:

- Frozen banana (sliced): 1
- Kale (remove stems and chop leaves): ¾ cup
- Almond milk: ¾ cup
- Almond butter: ¾ Tbsp.
- Cinnamon: 1/8 tsp.
- Nutmeg: 1/8 tsp.
- Ground ginger: 1/8 tsp.

XXXXXXXXXXXXXXXXXXXXXXXXXXXXXXXXX

Methods:

Combine all fruits, nuts and rest of the ingredients in one blender and blend them to make a smooth blend. Serve immediately!

Recipe 2: Cashew Cherry Smoothie

Nutritional Importance: This smoothie is really delicious with its sweet and soft texture. This smoothie is loaded with essential vitamins, nutrients, magnesium and various other minerals. It is good to reduce your blood pressure and improve health of your brain.

Preparation Time: 5 Minutes

Yield: 2 smoothies

List of Ingredients:

- Raw cashews: ½ cup
- Spinach (fresh leaves): 2 cups
- Cherries (frozen): ½ cup
- Banana (frozen): 2 medium
- Coconut milk (unsweetened): 2 cups
- Chia seeds: 2 Tbsp.
- Seed or nut butter: 2 Tbsp.

XXXXXXXXXXXXXXXXXXXXXXXXXXXXXXXXX

Methods:

Add all ingredients in a blender and process them for a few minutes to get a smooth and consistent blend. Enjoy cold smoothie!

Recipe 3: Strawberry and Pomegranate Smoothie

Nutritional Importance: This smoothie has lots of fuel for your body with antioxidants, polyphenols and all essential nutrients to improve your brain health and energize your body.

Preparation Time: 5 Minutes

Yield: 1 to 2 smoothies

List of Ingredients:

- Pomegranate juice: 1/3 cup
- Raw honey: 2 tsp.
- Frozen strawberries (unsweetened): ¾ cup
- Plain yogurt (fat-free): 2 Tbsp.
- Flaxseed oil: 1 Tbsp.
- Ice cubes: 4

xxxxxxxxxxxxxxxxxxxxxxxxxxxxxxxxxxx

Methods:

Take a small cup and whisk honey and pomegranate juice to dissolve honey.

Take a blender and blend yogurt, strawberries, ice cubes, pomegranate mixture, and oil. Process it for 2 minutes to get a smooth and thick blend. Pour into glasses and serve.

Recipe 4: Belly and Brain Soother

Nutritional Importance: Treat your brain and tummy at the same time with this papaya soother. Papaya is good for your tummy and almond is excellent for your brain.

Preparation Time: 5 Minutes

Yield: 2 smoothies

List of Ingredients:

- Papaya: 1 cup
- Coconut milk or yogurt: 1 cup
- Lime juice: ½ lime
- Honey: 1 Tbsp.
- Walnuts: 1 Tbsp.

XXXXXXXXXXXXXXXXXXXXXXXXXXXXXXXXXX

Methods:

Make a smooth blend of all ingredients in a blender and serve cold.

Recipe 5: Beet, Blueberry and Almond Smoothie

Nutritional Importance: Beets are good for your brain because these are high in folate, beta carotene, fiber, nitrates and phytonutrients. These can increase the flow of blood to your brain.

Preparation Time: 5 Minutes

Yield: 1 smoothie

List of Ingredients:

- Carrot juice (unsweetened): ½ cup
- Blueberries (fresh or frozen): ½ cup
- Raw beet (remove peels and grated): ½ cup
- Applesauce (unsweetened): ½ cup
- Whole almonds (unsalted): ½ cup
- Ice cubes: ½ cup
- Lime juice: ½ tsp.
- Ground ginger: 1 dash

xxxxxxxxxxxxxxxxxxxxxxxxxxxxxxxxxx

Methods:

Combine all fruits and rest of the ingredients in one blender and blend them to make a smooth blend. Serve immediately!

Chapter IV – Anti-aging and Beauty Smoothies

xxxxxxxxxxxxxxxxxxxxxxxxxxxxxxxxxxxx

If you want to increase your beauty and reduce anti-aging process naturally, you can get the advantage of these smoothies:

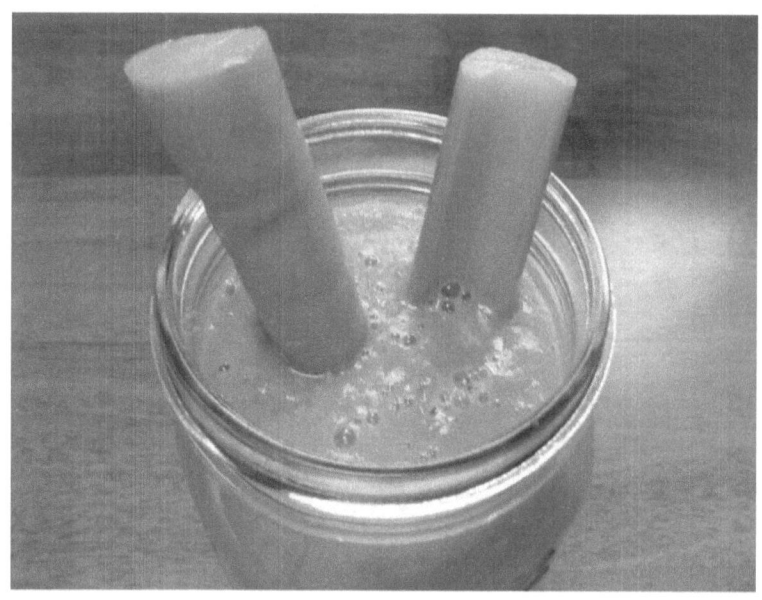

Recipe 1: Paradise Smoothie for Skin

Nutritional Importance: This smoothie is great to remove wrinkles, cleanse your skin and bring glow to your face. Vitamin C will improve elasticity of your skin and generates new cells.

Preparation Time: 5 Minutes

Yield: 2 smoothies

List of Ingredients:

- Ripe peach (slices): 1 medium
- Avocado (chopped): 2 Tbsp.
- Frozen strawberries (unsweetened): ½ cup
- Plain yogurt (fat-free): ¾ cup
- Pomegranate juice: 3 Tbsp.
- Grapeseed oil: 1 tsp.
- Vanilla extract: 1 tsp.

XXXXXXXXXXXXXXXXXXXXXXXXXXXXXXXXX

Methods:

Put each and every ingredient in a blender and blend them for one minute or more to blend everything. You should get a smooth mixture. Pour in glasses and serve chilled.

Recipe 2: Carrot and Kale Smoothie

Nutritional Importance: This smoothie is really healthy to improve elasticity and shine of your skin. It will be an amazing addition to your diet to get a healthy and fair skin.

Preparation Time: 5 Minutes

Yield: 2 smoothies

List of Ingredients:

- Kale (remove stems and chop only leaves): 1 cup
- Carrot (chopped): 1
- Green apple (remove core and chopped): 1
- Lemon juice: 1 to 2 Tbsp.
- Coconut water: 1 cup

XXXXXXXXXXXXXXXXXXXXXXXXXXXXXXXX

Methods:

Put all ingredients in a blender and blend everything well for a few minutes. You will get a smooth paste, pour into glasses and serve cold.

Recipe 3: Amazing Beauty Smoothie

Nutritional Importance: Antioxidants can help you to fight with stress and tension. Ingredients of this smoothie will help you to improve the texture and beauty of your skin.

Preparation Time: 5 Minutes

Yield: 2 smoothies

List of Ingredients:

- Frozen strawberries: ¼ cup
- Frozen blueberries: ½ cup
- Orange (remove pits and peels): 1
- Banana: 1 ripe
- Plain yogurt (fat-free): ½ cup
- Silken tofu: ½ cup
- Chai seeds: 2 Tbsp.
- Agave nectar: 1 tsp.

xxxxxxxxxxxxxxxxxxxxxxxxxxxxxxxxxx

Methods:

Take a blender, put all ingredients in this blender and blend them well to get a smooth drink. Enjoy cold and feel younger.

Recipe 4: Beauty Blast of Berries

Nutritional Importance: If you want to get a glowing and wrinkle free skin, this smoothie will be a right choice for you. Follow its simple and easy recipe:

Preparation Time: 5 Minutes

Yield: 2 smoothies

List of Ingredients:

- Blueberries: ¼ cup
- Strawberries: ¼ cup
- Raspberries: ¼ cup
- Kale: ¼ cup
- Almond milk: 1 cup
- Chia seeds: 1 tsp.
- Water: 1 cup (optional)
- Ice cubes: 3 to 4

xxxxxxxxxxxxxxxxxxxxxxxxxxxxxxxxxx

Methods:

Put all ingredients one-by-one in a blender and blend them to get a smooth mixture. You can add water to adjust its thickness. Serve immediately.

Note: If you are using frozen berries, there is no need to use ice because frozen berries will make your smoothie cold.

Recipe 5: Glowing Smoothie for Healthy Skin

Nutritional Importance: It is low in calories and high in fiber. This smoothie offers folate, vitamins and essential nutrients to improve your overall health.

Preparation Time: 5 Minutes

Yield: 2 smoothies

List of Ingredients:

- Spinach leaves: 1 cup
- Kale (chopped): 1 cup
- Seedless grapes (green): 1 cup
- Bartlett pear (remove seeds, core and stem):
- Orange (remove peels and quartered): 1
- Peeled Banana: 1
- Chia seeds: 1 tsp.
- Water: ½ cup
- Ice: 2 cups

xxxxxxxxxxxxxxxxxxxxxxxxxxxxxxxxxx

Methods:

Before making a smoothie, carefully wash kale and spinach. Now, place each and every ingredient in a blender and blend them for one minute to blend everything. This smoothie will taste really good and increase shine and health of your skin.

Chapter V – Diabetic Smoothies

xxxxxxxxxxxxxxxxxxxxxxxxxxxxxxxxxxx

If you are a diabetic patient, you can try these smoothies that are healthy and delicious. These smoothies are good for every diabetic patient:

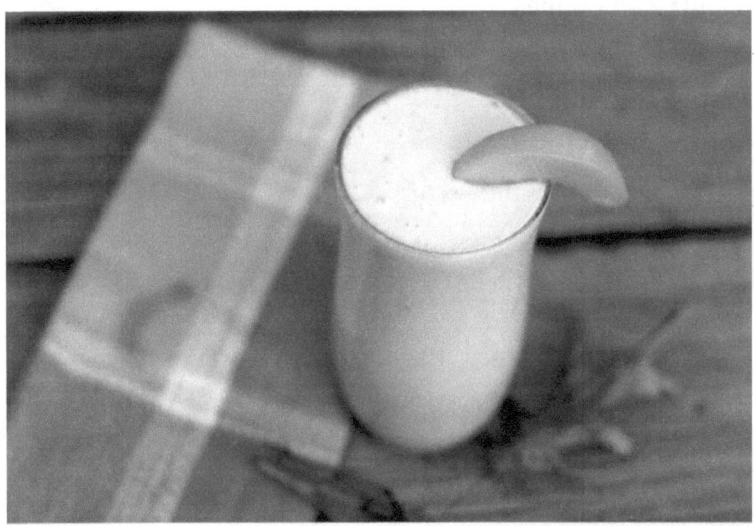

Recipe 1: Chia Seed and Spinach Smoothie

Nutritional Importance: This delicious smoothie is low in fat and high in zinc, protein, niacin, essential vitamins, thiamin, calcium, folate, phosphorus, copper and iron.

Preparation Time: 5 Minutes

Yield: 2 smoothies

List of Ingredients:

- Coconut milk: 1 cup
- Chia seeds: 2 Tbsp.
- Spinach: 1 cup
- Protein Powder: 1 scoop
- Ice cubes: 2

XXXXXXXXXXXXXXXXXXXXXXXXXXXXXXXXXX

Methods:

Add all ingredients in a blender and blend them to have a consistent and delicious smoothie. Serve immediately!

Recipe 2: Almond and Berry Smoothie

Nutritional Importance: Start your day with this refreshing smoothie because almond milk is low in carb and great for diabetic patients and people with lactose intolerance.

Preparation Time: 5 Minutes

Yield: 2 smoothies

List of Ingredients:

- Almond milk: 1 cup
- Peaches (frozen): 1 cup
- Strawberries (frozen): 1 cup
- Greek yogurt: 3.5 ounce

xxxxxxxxxxxxxxxxxxxxxxxxxxxxxxxx

Methods:

Blend all ingredients in one blender and make a smooth puree. Pour in glasses and serve immediately.

Recipe 3: Superfood Smoothie

Nutritional Importance: This smoothie is good for your external and internal body. You can enjoy this smoothie without worrying about your diabetes:

Preparation Time: 5 Minutes

Yield: 2 smoothies

List of Ingredients:

- Almond milk: ¾ cup
- Frozen blueberries: ½ cup
- Frozen strawberries: 1/3 cup
- Avocado (pitted and chopped): ½
- Spinach: 1 handful
- Flaxseed: 1 Tbsp.
- Chia seeds: 1 Tbsp.
- Protein powder: 1 scoop (optional)
- Green superfood: 1 scoop
- Ice cubes: 4

XXXXXXXXXXXXXXXXXXXXXXXXXXXXXXXXXX

Methods:

Blend all ingredients to make a consistent and smooth paste. This will be a delicious smoothie.

Recipe 4: Oatmeal Smoothie for Diabetes

Nutritional Importance: This smoothie will be a great source of fiber, calcium and potassium. It can reduce your blood pressure and improve your diabetic condition.

Preparation Time: 5 Minutes

Yield: 2 smoothies

List of Ingredients:

- Uncooked oats: 1 cup
- Banana: 2 frozen
- Skim milk: 3 cups
- Flaxseed (ground): 2 Tbsp.
- Coffee extract: 2 tsp.

xxxxxxxxxxxxxxxxxxxxxxxxxxxxxxxxxx

Methods:

Combine all above ingredients in a blender and blend them well. Pour this blend into glasses and enjoy!

Recipe 5: Peach Smoothie

Nutritional Importance: This smoothie is packed with potassium, manganese, zinc, copper, and dietary fiber. It is good to control your cholesterol and improve overall health.

Preparation Time: 5 Minutes

Yield: 2 smoothies

List of Ingredients:

- Fresh peach (pitted & chopped): 1
- Skim milk: ½ cup
- Vanilla yogurt: 4 ounce
- Ice cubes: 1 cup
- Ground cinnamon: As per taste

xxxxxxxxxxxxxxxxxxxxxxxxxxxxxxxxxxx

Methods:

Put milk, peach, ice and yogurt in one blender. Blend them for a few minutes to make a smooth paste. Turn off blender and scrape down all sides of the blender with a rubber spatula. Pour this mixture into two glasses and sprinkle cinnamon on each glass. Garnish with strawberry slices and serve cold smoothies.

Chapter VI – Tips and Tricks for Juicing and Blending

XXXXXXXXXXXXXXXXXXXXXXXXXXXXXXX

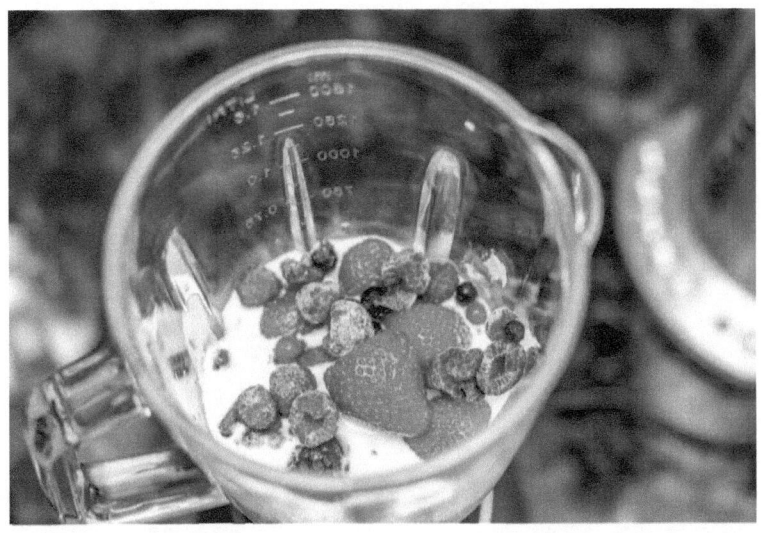

Juices and smoothies are really healthy for your body because they have lots of vitamins, minerals, and other healthy nutrients. You have to focus on the texture and combination of fruits and juices. Juicing extracts, a small amount of liquid from particular ingredients, such as herbs and leafy greens. You can blend these ingredients to make smoothies. Smoothies and juices are great in taste until something goes wrong. You shouldn't combine bitter and sour tastes together. You can get some optimal balances with practice and experimentation. There are a few things that will help you to enhance the taste of your juice:

(1) Simple Formula for Tasty Juice

You can enhance the taste of your juices with a few combinations that are given below. Some produce has spicy flavors, earthy, sweet or sour taste, but you should be careful while combining different fruits and vegetables. There are some famous ingredients that are organized as per their taste:

- Tart: Lemons and limes
- Sweet: Pears, apples, grapes, pineapples, melons, oranges, mangoes, kiwis, berries and grapes
- Roots: Carrots, beets, parsnips, and turnips
- Herbs: Basil, cilantro, mint and parsley
- Greens: Spinach, Kale, lettuce, arugula, chard, beet greens, mustard greens, dandelion, broccoli and sorrel
- High-yield: Celery, cucumbers, fennel, melons and tomatoes
- Spicy: Hot peppers and ginger (use sensibly)

Juices Together that you would like to Eat Together

People often sound confused for the combination of different fruits and vegetables, but there is a common sense to combine those fruits and vegetables that you would like to eat together. You can use a good quality juicer to extract the juices of fruits and vegetables. If you can make a good salad with your selected combination, you can select them to make juice. Keep it in mind that you can change the quantity and high-yield ingredients, such as celery or cucumber to fill your juice.

Balance High-Yield Ingredients with High-Potency Ingredients

You should balance cucumbers, apples, and celery because these are tsunamis for juicing. Mint and ginger can be a little bit bitter; therefore, be aware of the behavior of every ingredient in a juicer. You should try a reasonable balance between mellow ingredients and intense ones.

Adjust Taste Accordingly

You can adjust the taste of your juice accordingly by squeezing a lemon or adding an extra chunk of apple. You can increase or decrease apples and vegetables in juices as per your taste.

Peel or No to Peel

It doesn't matter to remove the skin of fruits and vegetables because both ways are good. Always buy organic vegetables and fruits to extract their juice with the skin. If your fruits and vegetables are grown on a farm, you should remove their peels because these are treated with pesticides. The peels may contain dangerous chemicals that are harmful to your health. You should peel the following produce:

(2) Waxed Produce

Kiwis

Citrus fruits (you should not peel, if you want a pure taste of oil and the bitterness of the fruit. Juice the whole thing will change the flavor)

Any ingredient where you doubt that the skin can affect the taste

You can remove the skin of any fruit that can affect the color of the final juice, such as the skin of cucumber should be removed in a watermelon juice

Leafy Greens

There are three essential flavors of leafy greens, such as lettuce, beet greens, kale, and chard are neutral flavors. Dandelion, arugula, and mustard are peppery flavors. You can easily deal neutral flavors, but the peppery flavor is impossible to hide, but you can make them the stars of the show with an excellent combination. Earthy greens require little more coaxing. Kale is found in many juices and smoothies, but lonely liquid kale may not taste good. You can prepare a blend of acid, herbs and kale along with lemon juice.

Consider Color

You should consider the colors of your juice, such as gray and brown juice should be tried without penchant or an opaque cup along with a lid for the grotesque. In green juices, apples and peers can be better than strawberries. You can juice a beet for its lovely color. In short, the color can be a trump card and will help you to determine the taste and the combination of juices.

(3) Shopping and Cleaning Tips

If you are going to buy fruits and vegetables, make sure to select organic produce. Carefully check the fruits and vegetables because these should be free from bruise and marks. If the color of vegetable is different than natural color, you should avoid it. You should carefully wash your fruits and vegetables before juicing them. It will be good to use soapy water to wash away any wax and chemical.

Tips to Get Maximum Juice

You can increase the yield from your ingredients by considering the speed of your juicer. If you want to extract the juices of green vegetables, you should tightly pack the greens and adjust them between harder ingredients, such as apple and cucumber. It will be good to use a slow speed for citrus, stone fruits, melons, berries and other similar fruits. Thoroughly wash your selected vegetables and cut them into small pieces to easily handle them in your juicer.

Store in Fridge

You should keep the juice for almost 24 to 48 hours in the fridge, while traveling. An airtight container is a good choice to secure juice, but always select a glass container or BPA-free plastic. Fill your container to the top to avoid oxygen from getting in and deplete the nutrients. Freezing is a good choice and you can thaw your juice in the refrigerator for almost 7 to 10 days. Always store your juices in dark and cold environments, away from light and heat.

(4) Tips to Buy Right Juicers and Blenders

Basically, three main types of juicers are available in the market, such as triturating, centrifugal and masticating. All machines have their own strengths and weaknesses. The basic difference is that the masticating juicers can chew, the centrifugal machine is for grinding and triturating is good to press produce. There are numerous juicing machines available in the market and it can be difficult for you to take a decision. There are a few tips for you to buy juicers:

Important Things to Check

Centrifugal and blender-style juicers have lots of competition and these two types are different from each other. Centrifugal has a rotating blade system to grind produce, but the blender-style juicers can leave the pulp in the juice. The centrifugal units can separate most of the pulp out of its juice. Blender-style and centrifugal units may add oxygen and heat to produce, and oxygen can subtract nutritional benefits. You can select any type of juicer as per your needs, but there are a few characteristics to consider:

Juicing Capabilities

The best juice maker can extract the maximum amount of juice because they have powerful motors to yield maximum juice. If you want to test a juicer to check its yield, make sure to select different types of fruits and vegetables. You can try lemons, kale, apple, beets, spinach, carrots, oranges, ginger and grapefruit to check the behavior of machine with different types of fruits. The basic purpose of juicing is to make the fruits and vegetables more palatable. Your selected juicer should help you to get the smoothest juices with less pulp.

Preparation and Cleaning

The best juicer should require little preparation and it should be simple to assemble. You can consider its parts, washing style, and size. Your selected machine should make less noise in the early morning. Check the built-in storage for cord and nonslip base to make it convenient.

Help and Support

The machine should have a long and strong body and their manufacturers should offer good warranties. The manufacturer should offer easy access to customer service representative. A fresh juicing routine will help you to add flavor and nutrients in your life. A glass of fresh juice will be more appetizing than raw produce. You should select a right juicer to start your day with a healthy habit that may last for your whole life.

Best Juicers Available in the Market

There are a few best juicers that are available in the market at different rates. A few best brands are mentioned below:

Centrifugal Juicer

Centrifugal juicers are famous for their speed and these can easily handle the hardest vegetables and fruits, with their cutting disks. These types of juicers have the ability to run at numerous thousand revolutions in one minute because they use centrifugal force to separate pulp and juice. This method is quick and convenient for juicing. These machines are not good for green vegetables. Centrifugal juicers are a bit noisy because of their fast speed. If you want quick juicing, these juicers are perfect options for you.

Horizontal Masticating Juicer

These types of juicers are typically good for green vegetables. If you want to juice a lot of spinach, cabbage, kale, herbs, wheatgrass and other similar vegetables, you can use these juicers. These machines are good for their dual performance because you can use them as a mincer or a grinder and you can also make baby foods, extrude pasta and nut butter. They are quieter and slower than versatile centrifugal juicers. You can get high-quality juice with a horizontal masticating juicer.

Vertical Masticating Juicers

These machines are better than traditional juicers with their compact and upright design. These juicers require little more care to avoid jamming issues and it is a little bit expensive than horizontal masticating juicers. They are good for quieter and good quality operations.

About the Author

Heston Brown is an accomplished chef and successful e-book author from Palo Alto California. After studying cooking at The New England Culinary Institute, Heston stopped briefly in Chicago where he was offered head chef at some of the city's most prestigious restaurants. Brown decide that he missed the rolling hills and sunny weather of California and moved back to his home state to open up his own catering company and give private cooking classes.

Heston lives in California with his beautiful wife of 18 years and his two daughters who also have aspirations to follow in their father's footsteps and pursue careers in the culinary arts. Brown is well known for his delicious fish and chicken dishes and teaches these recipes as well as many others to his students.

When Heston gave up his successful chef position in Chicago and moved back to California, a friend suggested he use the internet to share his recipes with the world and so he did! To date, Heston Brown has written over 1000 e-books that contain recipes, cooking tips, business strategies for catering companies and a self-help book he wrote from personal experience.

He claims his wife has been his inspiration throughout many of his endeavours and continues to be his partner in business as well as life. His greatest joy is having all three women in his life in the kitchen with him cooking their favourite meal while his favourite jazz music plays in the background.

Author's Afterthoughts

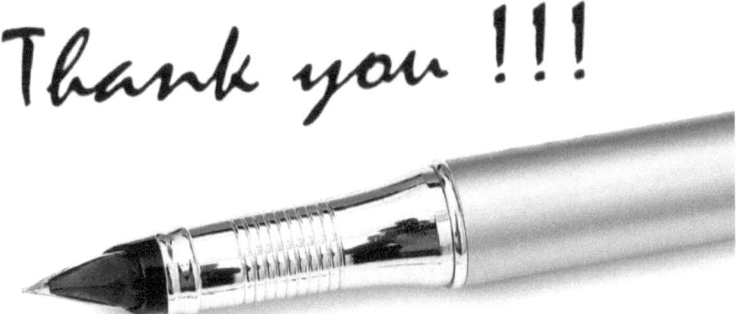

Thank you to all the readers who invested time and money into my book! I cherish every one of you and hope you took the same pleasure in reading it as I did in writing it.

Out of all of the books out there, you chose mine and for that I am truly grateful. It makes the effort worth it when I know my readers are enjoying my work from beginning to end.

Please take a few minutes to write an Amazon review so that others can benefit from your opinions and insight. Your review will help countless other readers make an informed choice

Thank you so much,

Heston Brown

www.ingramcontent.com/pod-product-compliance
Lightning Source LLC
Chambersburg PA
CBHW021244280526

45784CB00005B/2237